Sleep Soundly

Herbs for Restful Nights for the Whole Family

by
Meljay Turner

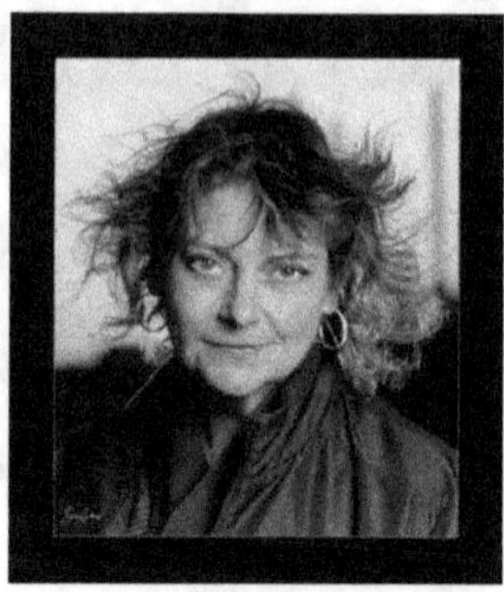

Meljay Turner is a loving and devoted mother of three, a thrill-seeker who has gripped the rails of the roller-coaster of life and is still screaming her joys as she speeds through the barrel rolls and loop-the-loops. Meljay has travelled the greatest adventure of life, motherhood, and now that the children are grown, she is on a new adventure, and what lies ahead we just never know for sure.

We all are on that train track of life, with many similarities in our lives, but ultimately what we do with that life is up to us. A rollercoaster of life however, just seemed one tracked, and life really is not like that, more like a train track with many stations, and many different trains we could get on. The question is what destination?

Author of motivational life experiences, life hacks, and business help, Meljay puts to paper the struggles and highs of life with hope that you are drawn into the stories, and find that you too, if you want to, choose a path of life that is of benefit to your family and friends, but ultimately you.

This book has been created with AI and human input.

All books can be found at www.meljayturner.com

Sleep Soundly Herbs for Restful Nights for the Whole Family

Proofreading, Typeset and Cover Design
by
Meljay Turner
with the aid of Artificial Intelligence
with Designrr in the
United Kingdom 2024.

Table Of Contents

Chapter 1: Introduction to Herbal Remedies for the Whole Family

Benefits of Using Herbs for Health and Wellness

Incorporating herbs into your family's health and wellness routine can have a multitude of benefits. From promoting better sleep to boosting mental clarity and focus, herbs are a natural and effective way to support your family's well-being.

One of the main advantages of using herbs for health is their natural properties. Unlike synthetic medications, herbs are derived from plants and are often less harsh on the body. This can be especially beneficial for children, as their developing bodies may be more sensitive to chemicals found in traditional medicines.

Herbs are also known for their versatility. They can be used in various forms such as teas, tinctures, or topical creams, making them easy to incorporate into your daily routine. For parents looking to address common ailments in children, herbs can provide gentle and effective relief for issues such as colic, teething pain, or cold symptoms.

When it comes to promoting better sleep for the whole family, herbs like chamomile, valerian, and lavender are known for their calming properties.

These herbs can help relax the body and mind, making it easier to drift off to sleep naturally.

In addition to physical health benefits, herbs can also be used for natural skincare and beauty. Herbs like aloe vera, calendula, and rosemary have been used for centuries to nourish and rejuvenate the skin, leaving you with a healthy and radiant complexion.

For those interested in growing their own herbs, herbal gardening tips can help you cultivate a thriving herb garden right at home. This not only gives you access to fresh and potent herbs but also allows you to connect with nature and enjoy the therapeutic benefits of gardening.

Overall, incorporating herbs into your family's health and wellness routine can provide numerous benefits for both the body and mind. Whether you're looking to improve sleep, support mental clarity, or simply promote overall well-being, herbs are a natural and effective solution for the whole family.

How Herbal Remedies Can Benefit the Entire Family

As parents, and I have three grown up children now, we always want what's best for our families, especially when it comes to their health and well-being. Herbal remedies have been used for centuries to treat various ailments and promote overall wellness, making them a great natural alternative for the entire family.

Using herbal remedies can benefit the whole family in numerous ways. For children, herbal remedies can be used to treat common ailments such as colds, coughs, and stomach-aches. Herbs like chamomile, ginger, and echinacea have been shown to be effective in boosting the immune system and alleviating symptoms of illness in children.

When it comes to promoting better sleep for the whole family, herbs like valerian, lavender, and passionflower can be used to help relax the mind and body, making it easier to fall asleep and stay asleep throughout the night. Incorporating these herbs into a bedtime routine can help create a peaceful and restful environment for everyone in the family.

Herbal remedies can also be used for natural skincare and beauty for the family. Herbs like aloe vera, calendula, and lavender have soothing and healing properties that can help treat skin conditions, promote healthy hair, and maintain a youthful appearance.

If you're interested in growing your own herbs at home, there are plenty of herbal gardening tips available to help you get started, I will be able to help you along the way too with different herbs I have found to grow well with minimal maintenance. Growing your own herbs not only ensures that you have a fresh supply on hand, but it also allows you to connect with nature and experience the therapeutic benefits of gardening. I used to grow herbs for the horses and had a small allotment area specifically for that, which was a wonderful experience being in nature.

In addition to physical health, herbal remedies can also promote mental clarity and focus for the whole family. Herbs like ginkgo biloba, rosemary, and peppermint have been shown to improve cognitive function and enhance memory, making them great options for busy parents and students alike.

Overall, incorporating herbal remedies into your family's routine can have a positive impact on everyone's health and well-being. Whether you're looking to treat common ailments, improve sleep quality, enhance beauty, or boost mental focus, there's an herb out there that can help you achieve your goals naturally and effectively.

Importance of Natural Remedies for Children

As parents, we all want to provide the best care for our children, especially when it comes to their health and well-being. In today's modern world, it can be easy to rely on over-the-counter medications and quick fixes for common childhood ailments. However, the importance of natural remedies for children cannot be overlooked.

Natural remedies offer a gentle and holistic approach to treating common childhood illnesses and promoting overall well-being. As a child my mother used herbal remedies rather than over the counter medications, so this is something that has always been with me through my life. Many herbs and plants have been used for centuries to alleviate symptoms of coughs, colds, fevers, and digestive issues in children. These natural remedies work with the body's own healing mechanisms to support the immune system and promote a faster recovery.

When it comes to promoting better sleep for the whole family, natural remedies can be a game-changer. Herbs like chamomile, lavender, and valerian root have been traditionally used to calm the mind and body, making it easier to drift into sleep. By incorporating these herbs into your bedtime routine, you can create a peaceful environment that promotes restful nights for both you and your children.

In addition to supporting physical health, natural remedies can also be beneficial for promoting mental clarity and focus in children. Herbs like ginkgo biloba, bacopa, and rosemary have been shown to improve cognitive function and enhance memory. By incorporating these herbs into your family's daily routine, you can support your children's learning and development in a natural and sustainable way.

Overall, the importance of natural remedies for children cannot be overstated. By incorporating herbs and plants into your lifestyle, you can help promote better health, improved sleep, and enhanced mental clarity for the whole family. So why not give natural remedies a try and see the positive impact they can have on your children's well-being?

Chapter 2: Herbs for Promoting Better Sleep for the Whole Family

Lavender: Nature's Calming Herb

Lavender is not only a beautiful and fragrant herb, but it also holds powerful calming properties that can benefit the whole family. Whether you are struggling with insomnia, restless children, or just need a little help winding down at the end of a long day, lavender can be a natural solution to promote better sleep and relaxation.

For parents looking for natural remedies to help their children sleep soundly, lavender can be a gentle and safe option. A few drops of lavender essential oil on a pillow or in a di user can create a soothing environment that promotes restful sleep. Lavender can also be added to a warm bath before bedtime to help children relax and unwind before bed.

In addition to its sleep-inducing properties, lavender can also be used to promote mental clarity and focus for the whole family. The calming scent of lavender has been shown to reduce stress and anxiety, allowing for improved concentration and productivity. Whether you are studying for exams or just trying to stay focused during a busy day, a whisp of lavender can help clear your mind and boost your mental clarity.

For parents interested in incorporating lavender into their daily routines, consider growing your own lavender plants at home. Lavender is relatively easy to grow and can thrive in a variety of climates. By cultivating your own lavender plants, you can have a fresh supply of this calming herb at your fingertips whenever you need it.

Overall, lavender is a versatile and beneficial herb that can improve the quality of sleep for the whole family, promote mental clarity and focus, and provide natural skincare and beauty benefits. Consider incorporating lavender into your daily routine to enjoy its calming and soothing effects.

Chamomile: The Ultimate Relaxation Herb

Chamomile is a well-known herb that has been used for centuries as a natural remedy for promoting relaxation and better sleep. This gentle herb is not only safe for adults but also for children, making it the ultimate relaxation herb for the whole family.

For parents looking for a natural solution to help their children wind down after a long day, chamomile can be a game-changer. This herb is known for its calming properties, which can help soothe restless minds and bodies, making it easier for both children and adults to fall asleep and stay asleep throughout the night.

Chamomile can be consumed in various forms, such as herbal tea, capsules, or even as an essential oil for aromatherapy. A warm cup of chamomile tea before bedtime can work wonders in promoting relaxation and preparing the body for a restful night's sleep. For children who may have trouble winding down, a few drops of chamomile essential oil in a di user can create a calming atmosphere in their bedroom.

In addition to its relaxation benefits, chamomile also has natural skincare and beauty properties that can benefit the whole family. It can help soothe irritated skin, reduce inflammation, and even promote a healthy complexion when used in skincare products or as a gentle toner.

For parents interested in growing their own herbs at home, chamomile is a great option for a beginner's herbal garden. This low-maintenance herb thrives in sunny locations and can be easily grown in containers or directly in the ground.

Overall, chamomile is truly the ultimate relaxation herb for the whole family, offering a natural solution for promoting better sleep, skincare, and mental clarity. Incorporating chamomile into your daily routine can help create a peaceful and restful environment for the entire family to enjoy.

Valerian Root: A Natural Sleep Aid

As parents, we all know the struggle of trying to get a good night's sleep when our little ones are restless. Valerian root, a natural sleep aid, may be the solution you've been looking for to help the whole family get the rest they need.

Valerian root has been used for centuries as a remedy for insomnia and other sleep disorders. It works by increasing the levels of a neurotransmitter called GABA in the brain, which helps to calm the nervous system and promote relaxation. This can make it easier to fall asleep and stay asleep throughout the night.

One of the great things about valerian root is that it is safe for children to use, making it a fantastic option for parents looking for natural remedies for their little ones. Whether your child is having trouble falling asleep at night or is waking up frequently, valerian root may be just what they need to get the restful sleep they deserve.

In addition to its sleep-inducing properties, valerian root also has other health benefits. It can help to reduce anxiety and stress, promote mental clarity and focus, and even improve the overall quality of your skin and hair. By incorporating valerian root into your family's daily routine, you can experience the many benefits that this powerful herb has to offer.

If you're interested in trying valerian root as a natural sleep aid for your family, consider growing your own herb garden at home. Valerian root is relatively easy to grow and can thrive in a variety of climates. By having a fresh supply of valerian root on hand, you can ensure that your family always has access to this wonderful herb whenever they need it.

In conclusion, valerian root is a safe and effective natural sleep aid that can benefit the whole family. Consider adding this powerful herb to your family's wellness routine and enjoy the restful nights that you've been dreaming of.

Passionflower: Promoting Restful Nights

Passionflower, of the Passifloraceae family group, is a beautiful and delicate herb that has been used for centuries to promote restful nights and alleviate anxiety and stress. For parents looking for natural solutions to help their families get better sleep, passionflower may just be the herb they've been looking for.

Passionflower is rich in compounds that have a calming effect on the nervous system, making it an excellent choice for promoting relaxation and improving sleep quality. Whether you or your children struggle with falling asleep, staying asleep, or experience restless nights, passionflower can help soothe the mind and body to promote a deeper and more restful sleep.

For children who may have trouble winding down before bedtime, a cup of passionflower tea or a few drops of passionflower tincture can help create a calming bedtime routine. For parents who have trouble quieting their minds after a long day, passionflower can provide relief from racing thoughts and help promote a sense of tranquillity and peace.

In addition to its sleep-inducing properties, passionflower also offers a range of other benefits for the whole family. It can help improve mental clarity and focus, making it a great herb for students or parents who need a little extra brainpower during the day. Passionflower can also be used in natural skincare and beauty products to promote healthy, glowing skin for the whole family.

For those interested in growing their own herbs at home, passionflower is a relatively easy herb to cultivate and can thrive in a variety of climates. Whether you choose to grow it in a garden or in a pot on your windowsill, having a fresh supply of passionflower on hand can ensure that you always have access to its sleep-promoting and calming benefits.

Overall, passionflower is a versatile and effective herb that can benefit the whole family. By incorporating it into your daily routine, you can enjoy more restful nights, improved mental clarity, and a sense of calm and relaxation that will benefit both you and your loved ones.

Chapter 3: Herbal Remedies for Children's Common Ailments

Echinacea: Boosting Immunity in Kids

As parents, we all want our children to be healthy and strong, especially when it comes to fighting common illnesses. Echinacea is a powerful herb that has been used for centuries to boost the immune system and help ward o colds, u, and other common ailments in children.

One of the key benefits of echinacea is its ability to stimulate the production of white blood cells, which are the body's first line of defence against infections. By incorporating echinacea into your child's daily routine, you can help strengthen their immune system and reduce their risk of getting sick.

Echinacea can be taken in a variety of forms, including teas, tinctures, and supplements. For children who may not enjoy the taste of echinacea tea, there are also kid-friendly chewable tablets available. It's important to follow the recommended dosage guidelines for children to ensure they are getting the right amount of this powerful herb.

In addition to boosting immunity, echinacea can also help reduce the severity and duration of colds and u symptoms in children. By giving your child echinacea at the first sign of illness, you can help them recover more quickly and get back to their normal routine.

Overall, echinacea is a safe and effective herb for boosting immunity in kids. By incorporating this powerful herb into your child's daily routine, you can help keep them healthy and strong all year round.

Ginger: Soothing Upset Stomachs

As parents, we all know the struggle of dealing with upset stomachs in our children. Whether it's from eating too much junk food, feeling anxious, or just a general tummy ache, it can be challenging to find a natural remedy that actually works. This is where ginger comes in.

Ginger has long been used as a natural remedy for upset stomachs, nausea, and indigestion. It is known for its soothing properties that can help calm an upset stomach and promote digestion. Ginger contains compounds that can help reduce inflammation in the stomach and intestines, making it an effective solution for a range of digestive issues.

One of the easiest ways to use ginger for upset stomachs is by making a simple ginger tea. Simply steep a few slices of fresh ginger in hot water for a few minutes, then strain and sweeten with honey if desired. This warm and comforting tea can help relax the stomach muscles and ease any discomfort your child may be feeling.

You can also try giving your child ginger candies or chews made with real ginger extract. These can be a convenient and tasty way to help soothe their stomach while on the go or when they're not feeling up to drinking tea.

Overall, incorporating ginger into your family's herbal remedies toolkit can be a game-changer when it comes to soothing upset stomachs. Its natural properties make it a safe and effective option for children and adults alike, providing relief without the need for harsh chemicals or medications. So the next time your little one is feeling under the weather, reach for some ginger and let its soothing properties work their magic.

Peppermint: Relieving Digestive Discomfort

Peppermint has long been regarded as a powerful herb for relieving digestive discomfort in both adults and children. This versatile herb can be used in various forms, such as tea, essential oil, or as a topical balm, to help alleviate symptoms of indigestion, bloating, gas, and nausea.

For parents looking for natural remedies to soothe their child's upset stomach, peppermint is a safe and effective option. Its soothing properties can help alleviate discomfort and promote healthy digestion without the need for over-the-counter medications. Simply steeping a few fresh peppermint leaves in hot water to make a calming tea can provide quick relief for an upset tummy.

Peppermint essential oil can also be used topically to ease digestive discomfort. Simply dilute a few drops of peppermint oil with a carrier oil, such as coconut or almond oil, and gently massage it onto the abdomen in a clockwise motion. The cooling sensation of the peppermint oil can help relax the muscles in the digestive tract and ease bloating and gas.

In addition to its digestive benefits, peppermint can also promote better sleep for the whole family. Its calming properties can help relax the mind and body, making it easier to fall asleep and stay asleep throughout the night. Adding a few drops of peppermint essential oil to a di user in the bedroom can create a soothing atmosphere that promotes restful sleep for both adults and children.

Overall, peppermint is a versatile herb that can be a valuable addition to any family's herbal medicine cabinet. Whether you're looking to ease digestive discomfort, promote better sleep, or simply enjoy the refreshing aroma of peppermint, this herb has something to o er for everyone in the family.

Calendula: Healing Skin Irritations

Calendula, also known as marigold, is a powerful herb that has been used for centuries to heal skin irritations. This vibrant orange flower is not only beautiful to look at but also contains potent healing properties that make it a must-have in any herbal medicine cabinet.

For parents looking for natural remedies to soothe their children's skin ailments, calendula is a fantastic option. Whether it's a bug bite, diaper rash, eczema, or minor cuts and scrapes, calendula can help speed up the healing process and reduce inflammation. Its anti-inflammatory and antiseptic properties make it ideal for treating a variety of skin conditions without the use of harsh chemicals or synthetic ingredients.

In addition to its healing properties, calendula can also promote better sleep for the whole family. When used in herbal teas or tinctures, calendula can help calm the nervous system and promote relaxation, making it easier for both parents and children to drift o into a restful slumber.

For parents interested in incorporating calendula into their family's skincare routine, this versatile herb can be used in a variety of ways. Calendula-infused oils and salves can be applied topically to soothe dry, irritated skin or used as a natural alternative to traditional skincare products.

Growing calendula at home is also easy and rewarding. This resilient herb thrives in sunny locations and can be grown in containers or garden beds.

Harvesting and drying calendula flowers is a simple process that allows parents to have a fresh supply of this healing herb on hand whenever it's needed.

In conclusion, calendula is a versatile herb with a wide range of benefits for the whole family. From healing skin irritations to promoting better sleep, calendula is a valuable addition to any herbal medicine cabinet.

Chapter 4: Herbs for Natural Skincare and Beauty for the Family

Aloe Vera: Nature's Skin Soother

Aloe Vera is a versatile plant that has been used for centuries for its healing properties, especially when it comes to skincare. For parents looking for natural remedies to soothe their children's skin, Aloe Vera is a must-have in the herbal medicine cabinet.

This succulent plant is known for its cooling and moisturizing effects, making it perfect for treating sunburns, rashes, and other skin irritations that children may encounter. Its anti-inflammatory and antibacterial properties help to reduce redness and swelling, while promoting faster healing of damaged skin.

To use Aloe Vera for skin soothing purposes, simply break o a leaf from the plant and apply the gel-like substance directly onto the affected area. For added relief, you can also mix Aloe Vera gel with other calming herbs like chamomile or lavender to create a gentle skin ointment.

In addition to its skin-soothing benefits, Aloe Vera can also be incorporated into your family's skincare routine for overall health and beauty. Its hydrating properties make it an excellent natural moisturizer, helping to keep skin soft and supple. You can also use Aloe Vera gel as a gentle cleanser or facial mask to rejuvenate tired skin.

For parents interested in growing their own Aloe Vera plant at home, it's important to provide plenty of sunlight and well-draining soil. Aloe Vera is a low-maintenance plant that thrives in warm and dry conditions, making it a perfect addition to any herb garden.

In conclusion, Aloe Vera is a valuable herb for promoting healthy skin and overall well-being for the whole family. Its natural healing properties make it a go-to remedy for common skin ailments, while also offering beauty benefits for a glowing complexion. Consider adding Aloe Vera to your herbal medicine cabinet and skincare routine for a natural approach to health and wellness.

Rosemary: Stimulating Hair Growth

Rosemary is not just a delicious herb to add to your cooking; it also has amazing benefits for promoting hair growth and scalp health. For parents looking for natural remedies to help their children grow strong and healthy hair, rosemary is a great option.

Rosemary has been used for centuries in traditional medicine for its ability to stimulate hair follicles and improve circulation to the scalp. This increase in blood ow can promote hair growth and prevent hair loss. Rosemary oil can be massaged into the scalp to nourish the hair follicles and promote healthy hair growth.

In addition to stimulating hair growth, rosemary has antibacterial and anti-inflammatory properties that can help soothe an irritated scalp and reduce dandruff. This makes it a great option for children who may be struggling with scalp issues.

To use rosemary for stimulating hair growth, you can create a simple hair rinse by steeping fresh or dried rosemary in hot water and allowing it to cool. After shampooing, pour the rosemary rinse over your child's hair and scalp, massaging it in gently. Leave it on for a few minutes before rinsing it out.

For a more concentrated treatment, you can mix a few drops of rosemary essential oil with a carrier oil like coconut or olive oil and massage it into the scalp. Leave it on for at least 30 minutes before washing it out.

By incorporating rosemary into your hair care routine, you can help promote healthy hair growth for your children in a natural and effective way.

Tea Tree Oil: Fighting Acne Naturally

Tea tree oil is a powerful natural remedy that can help combat acne in both children and adults. Acne is a common skin condition that can be frustrating and embarrassing, especially for teenagers. The antibacterial and anti-inflammatory properties of tea tree oil make it an effective treatment for acne, helping to reduce redness and swelling while killing the bacteria that cause breakouts.

When using tea tree oil for acne, it is important to dilute it with a carrier oil such as jojoba or coconut oil to avoid irritation. Simply mix a few drops of tea tree oil with your chosen carrier oil and apply it to the affected areas of the skin. You can also add a few drops of tea tree oil to your regular face wash or moisturizer for an added boost.

Tea tree oil can also be used as a spot treatment for individual pimples. Simply dab a small amount of diluted tea tree oil onto the pimple and leave it on overnight. The antibacterial properties of the oil will help to dry out the pimple and reduce inflammation.

In addition to its acne-fighting properties, tea tree oil can also help to promote clearer, healthier skin overall. Its antiseptic properties can help to prevent future breakouts, while its anti-inflammatory properties can help to soothe irritated skin.

By incorporating tea tree oil into your family's skincare routine, you can help to naturally combat acne and promote clearer, healthier skin for the whole family. Say goodbye to harsh chemical treatments and hello to the power of tea tree oil for fighting acne naturally.

Nettle: Improving Skin Health

Nettle, also known as stinging nettle, is a powerful herb that offers a wide range of benefits for the entire family. While it is commonly known for its ability to promote better sleep and mental clarity, nettle also has fantastic properties when it comes to improving skin health.

For parents looking for natural skincare solutions for their children, nettle is a great option. It is rich in antioxidants, which help protect the skin from damage caused by free radicals. This can help prevent premature aging and keep the skin looking youthful and healthy.

Nettle also has anti-inflammatory properties, making it an excellent choice for soothing irritated skin conditions such as eczema or insect bites. Its natural astringent properties can help tighten pores and reduce excess oil production, making it an ideal ingredient for those with oily or acne-prone skin.

To incorporate nettle into your family's skincare routine, you can make a simple nettle-infused oil or tea to use as a toner or moisturizer. You can also find skincare products that contain nettle extract, such as creams, lotions, and serums.

In addition to its skincare benefits, nettle is also a great herb to include in your family's diet. You can easily grow nettle at home in your herb garden and use it in soups, salads, and teas. By incorporating nettle into your family's daily routine, you can enjoy its many health benefits, including improved skin health.

Chapter 5: Herbal Gardening Tips for Growing Herbs at Home

Choosing the Right Herbs for Your Family's Needs

Choosing the right herbs for your family's needs can be a daunting task, especially with the wide variety of options available. However, with a little knowledge and research, you can find the perfect herbs to address your family's special needs.

When it comes to selecting herbs for your family, it's important to consider their individual health concerns and preferences. For children, gentle herbs like chamomile and lavender can be excellent choices for promoting relaxation and restful sleep. These herbs can also be used to alleviate common childhood ailments such as colic, teething pain, and anxiety.

For promoting better sleep for the whole family, herbs like valerian root, passionflower, and lemon balm can be helpful in calming the mind and body before bedtime. These herbs can be taken as teas, tinctures, or essential oils to promote a restful night's sleep for everyone in the household.

If you're interested in incorporating herbs into your family's skincare routine, herbs like calendula, chamomile, and lavender can be used to soothe and heal the skin naturally. These herbs can be infused into oils, creams, and lotions to promote healthy, radiant skin for the whole family.

For those looking to improve mental clarity and focus, herbs like ginkgo biloba, rosemary, and peppermint can be beneficial for enhancing cognitive function and concentration. These herbs can be taken as supplements, teas, or added to meals to support mental clarity and focus for parents and children alike.

By taking the time to research and choose the right herbs for your family's needs, you can create a natural and holistic approach to health and wellness that will benefit everyone in the household. Remember to consult with a healthcare professional or herbalist before starting any new herbal regimen, especially for children or those with existing health conditions, especially if you are on medication.

Creating a Family-Friendly Herb Garden

As parents, we are always looking for ways to improve the health and well-being of our families. One way to do this is by creating a family-friendly herb garden right in your own backyard. Not only will this provide you with fresh herbs for cooking and herbal remedies, but it can also be a fun and educational project for the whole family to enjoy.

When planning your herb garden, consider the special needs of your family. Are you looking to grow herbs for cooking, herbal remedies for common ailments, or herbs for promoting better sleep and mental clarity? By tailoring your herb garden to your family's special needs, you can ensure that you are growing the herbs that will be most beneficial to your loved ones.

For families with young children, consider growing herbs that are safe and gentle enough for their delicate systems. Herbs like chamomile, lavender, and lemon balm are known for their calming properties and can be used to promote better sleep and reduce anxiety in both children and adults.

To promote mental clarity and focus for the whole family, consider growing herbs like rosemary, peppermint, and sage. These herbs can help improve cognitive function and concentration, making them ideal for students or anyone looking to boost their brainpower.

By incorporating a variety of herbs into your family-friendly herb garden, you can create a holistic approach to health and wellness for your loved ones. Not only will you have a fresh and convenient supply of herbs at your fingertips, but you will also be teaching your children the importance of self-care and natural remedies. So roll up your sleeves, grab your gardening tools, and get ready to create a family-friendly herb garden that will benefit your entire household.

Tips for Growing Herbs Indoors

As parents, we often strive to create a safe and healthy environment for our families. One way to achieve this is by incorporating herbs into our daily lives. Growing herbs indoors is a great way to have access to fresh, organic herbs all year round. Here are some tips for successfully growing herbs indoors:

1. Choose the right location: Herbs need plenty of sunlight to thrive. Place your indoor herb garden in a sunny spot, such as a windowsill or balcony, where they can get at least 6-8 hours of sunlight per day.

2. Use the right containers: Make sure your herb pots have good drainage to prevent waterlogging. Choose pots with drainage holes at the bottom and use a well-draining potting mix to ensure your herbs' roots don't rot.

3. Water your herbs properly: Herbs like to be watered thoroughly but infrequently. Allow the top inch of soil to dry out before watering

again. Overwatering can lead to root rot, so be mindful of how much water your herbs are receiving.

4.   Provide proper ventilation: Indoor plants can be prone to pests and diseases due to lack of air flow. Make sure to provide proper ventilation by opening windows or using a fan to keep the air circulating around your herbs.

5.   Harvest regularly: Regularly harvesting your herbs will encourage new growth and prevent them from becoming leggy. Use sharp scissors to snip off the top few inches of each stem, being careful not to remove more than a third of the plant at any one time.

By following these tips, you can successfully grow a thriving indoor herb garden that will not only provide you with fresh herbs for cooking and natural remedies but also promote better sleep, mental clarity, and focus for the whole family. Happy gardening!

Harvesting and Preserving Your Homegrown Herbs

Harvesting and preserving your homegrown herbs is a rewarding and essential part of incorporating herbal remedies into your family's daily routine. Not only does it ensure that you have a fresh supply of herbs on hand whenever you need them, but it also allows you to maintain the potency and effectiveness of the herbs.

When it comes to harvesting your herbs, the best time to do so is in the morning after the dew has dried but before the sun is at its peak. This is when the essential oils in the herbs are at their highest concentration, making them more potent. Use sharp shears or scissors to cut the herbs, being careful not to damage the plant itself. It's important to only harvest what you need, as over-harvesting can weaken the plant and decrease its ability to produce more herbs in the future.

Once you have harvested your herbs, there are several methods you can use to preserve them for future use. One popular method is drying herbs by hanging them upside down in a cool, dry place with good air circulation. You can also dry herbs by laying them out on a clean, dry surface or using a dehydrator. Another option is to freeze herbs in ice cube trays with water or oil for easy use in cooking or herbal remedies.

By taking the time to harvest and preserve your homegrown herbs, you can ensure that your family has access to fresh, potent herbs whenever they are needed. Whether you are using herbs for promoting better sleep, treating common ailments in children, or simply enhancing the beauty and mental clarity of your family, having a well-stocked supply of herbs is essential for a natural and holistic approach to health and wellness.

Chapter 6: Herbs for Promoting Mental Clarity and Focus for the Family

Ginkgo Biloba: Enhancing Cognitive Function

Ginkgo Biloba is a powerful herb known for its ability to enhance cognitive function, making it a valuable addition to any family's herbal medicine cabinet. This ancient herb has been used for centuries in traditional medicine to improve memory, focus, and overall brain health.

For parents looking to support their children's cognitive development, Ginkgo Biloba can be a safe and natural option. By increasing blood flow to the brain, this herb can help improve attention span, concentration, and mental clarity in children of all ages. Whether your child is struggling in school or simply needs a little extra support in staying focused, Ginkgo Biloba may be the solution you've been looking for.

In addition to its cognitive benefits, Ginkgo Biloba is also known for its ability to promote better sleep for the whole family. By calming the mind and reducing stress and anxiety, this herb can help both children and parents unwind at the end of a long day and enjoy a restful night's sleep. Incorporating Ginkgo Biloba into your family's bedtime routine may be just the thing you need to ensure everyone gets the quality rest they deserve.

Whether you're looking for ways to support your family's mental clarity and focus or simply improve their overall well-being, Ginkgo Biloba is a versatile herb that can benefit everyone. Consider adding this powerful herb to your family's daily routine and experience the positive effects it can have on your cognitive function and sleep quality.

Ginseng: Improving Mental Alertness

Ginseng, a powerful herb known for its ability to improve mental alertness, can be a valuable addition to your family's herbal remedies. As parents, we often find ourselves juggling multiple tasks and responsibilities while trying to maintain our mental focus and clarity. Ginseng can help support our cognitive function and enhance our ability to stay sharp and alert throughout the day.

Ginseng is believed to work by increasing blood flow to the brain, which can help improve memory, concentration, and overall cognitive function. This can be particularly beneficial for children who may struggle with focus or attention issues at school. By incorporating ginseng into your family's daily routine, you can help support your children's academic performance and mental well-being.

In addition to its cognitive benefits, ginseng is also known for its energizing properties. This can be especially helpful for parents who often feel drained and fatigued from the demands of daily life. By taking ginseng regularly, you may experience a boost in energy levels that can help you tackle your to-do list with ease.

When it comes to promoting better sleep for the whole family, ginseng can also play a role. By improving mental alertness during the day, ginseng can help regulate your sleep-wake cycle and promote restful nights for both parents and children alike.

Incorporating ginseng into your family's herbal remedies can have a positive impact on your mental clarity, focus, and overall well-being. Consider adding this powerful herb to your daily routine to experience the benefits for yourself.

Lemon Balm: Calming the Mind

Lemon balm, is a versatile herb that has been used for centuries to promote relaxation and calmness. In this subchapter, we will explore the benefits of lemon balm for calming the mind and improving sleep for the whole family.

For parents looking for natural remedies to help their children unwind and relax before bedtime, lemon balm is a great option. This herb has mild sedative properties that can help soothe restless minds and promote a sense of calm. Whether your child is struggling with anxiety, stress, or simply having trouble winding down at the end of the day, a cup of lemon balm tea or a few drops of lemon balm essential oil in a diffuser can make a world of difference.

But lemon balm isn't just for children – parents can benefit from its calming properties as well. Whether you're dealing with the stresses of work, family, or everyday life, incorporating lemon balm into your daily routine can help you relax and unwind, allowing you to get a better night's sleep and wake up feeling refreshed and rejuvenated.

In addition to its calming effects, lemon balm is also known for its ability to promote mental clarity and focus. By reducing stress and anxiety, lemon balm can help improve cognitive function and concentration, making it an ideal herb for parents who need to stay sharp and focused throughout the day.

Whether you're looking to improve your family's sleep, reduce stress and anxiety, or simply promote a sense of calm and relaxation, lemon balm is a versatile herb that can benefit the whole family. Consider adding this herb to your herbal remedy toolkit and enjoy the many benefits it has to offer.

Gotu Kola: Boosting Brain Power

In today's fast-paced world, parents are constantly juggling work, household responsibilities, and taking care of their children. This can lead to stress, fatigue, and a lack of mental clarity. However, there is a natural solution that can help boost brain power and promote mental focus for the whole family - Gotu Kola.

Gotu Kola is a powerful herb known for its ability to improve cognitive function, enhance memory, and increase mental clarity. It has been used for centuries in traditional medicine to improve brain health and support overall well-being. For parents looking for a natural way to enhance their brain power, Gotu Kola is a great option.

One of the key benefits of Gotu Kola is its ability to improve blood circulation to the brain, which can help enhance cognitive function and mental focus. By increasing oxygen and nutrients to the brain, Gotu Kola can help improve memory, concentration, and overall brain function. This can be especially beneficial for parents who are looking to stay sharp and focused throughout the day.

In addition to its cognitive benefits, Gotu Kola also has calming properties that can help reduce stress and anxiety. This can be particularly helpful for parents who are feeling overwhelmed and need a natural way to relax and unwind. By incorporating Gotu Kola into their daily routine, parents can experience improved mental clarity, reduced stress, and enhanced overall wellbeing.

In conclusion, Gotu Kola is a powerful herb that can help boost brain power and promote mental focus for the whole family. By incorporating this natural remedy into their daily routine, parents can experience improved cognitive function, enhanced memory, and reduced stress. Give Gotu Kola a try and see the positive impact it can have on your family's mental clarity and focus.

Chapter 7: Conclusion

Incorporating Herbal Remedies into Your Family's Daily Routine

As parents, we always want what is best for our families. One way to promote overall health and well-being in your household is by incorporating herbal remedies into your daily routine. These natural remedies have been used for centuries to treat common ailments, promote better sleep, improve mental clarity, and enhance beauty.

For children's common ailments, herbs like chamomile, ginger, and echinacea can be used to boost their immune system and alleviate symptoms of colds, flu, and digestive issues. These herbs can easily be incorporated into teas, tinctures, or even added to meals for a natural and effective remedy.

When it comes to promoting better sleep for the whole family, herbs like valerian root, passionflower, and lavender can help calm the mind and body, making it easier to fall asleep and stay asleep throughout the night. Creating a relaxing bedtime routine that includes herbal teas or aromatherapy with essential oils can significantly improve the quality of sleep for everyone in your household.

For natural skincare and beauty, herbs like aloe vera, calendula, and rosemary have antibacterial and anti-inflammatory properties that can help soothe and heal the skin. These herbs can be used in homemade skincare products like lotions, creams, and masks to promote healthy and glowing skin for the whole family.

If you are interested in growing your herbs at home, consider starting a herbal garden with plants like mint, basil, and thyme. Not only will you have access to fresh herbs for your remedies, but gardening can also be a therapeutic and rewarding activity for the whole family.

Incorporating herbal remedies into your family's daily routine can have numerous benefits for everyone's health and well-being. By exploring the world of herbs and their natural healing properties, you can create a holistic approach to wellness that will benefit your family for years to come.

Tips for Finding and Using Quality Herbs

In today's fast-paced world, finding ways to promote restful nights for the whole family can be a challenge. One effective solution that many parents are turning to is the use of herbs. Herbs have been used for centuries to promote relaxation, improve sleep quality, and even enhance mental clarity and focus. If you are interested in incorporating herbs into your family's daily routine, here are some tips for finding and using quality herbs.

1.   Research reputable sources: When looking for herbs, it is important to purchase them from reputable sources. Look for companies that specialize in herbal remedies and have a good reputation for quality and purity.

2.   Choose organic whenever possible: Organic herbs are grown without the use of synthetic pesticides or fertilizers, making them a healthier option for your family. Look for herbs that are certified organic to ensure that you are getting the best quality product.

3.   Start with the basics: If you are new to using herbs, start with some of the more common varieties such as chamomile, lavender, or valerian. These herbs are known for their calming and sleep-inducing properties and

can be a great place to start for promoting better sleep for the whole family.

4.   Consult with a professional: If you are unsure about which herbs to use or how to use them safely, consider consulting with a professional herbalist. They can provide guidance on which herbs are best suited for your family's needs and how to use them effectively.

5.   Experiment with different methods: Herbs can be used in a variety of ways, including teas, tinctures, capsules, and essential oils. Experiment with different methods to see which works best for your family and their individual preferences.

By following these tips for finding and using quality herbs, you can help promote restful nights and overall well-being for your family. Incorporating herbs into your daily routine can be a natural and effective way to improve sleep quality, promote mental clarity, and enhance overall health and wellness for the whole family.

Embracing a Natural Lifestyle for Better Health and Wellness

In today's fast-paced world, it can be easy to overlook the importance of embracing a natural lifestyle for better health and wellness. As parents, it is crucial to prioritize the well-being of the entire family, and one way to do so is by incorporating herbs into your daily routine.

Herbs have been used for centuries as natural remedies for a wide range of ailments, and they can be especially beneficial for children. From soothing upset stomachs to easing the symptoms of a cold, herbs offer a gentle and effective alternative to traditional medicine. By learning about the various herbs that can help with common childhood ailments, parents can empower themselves to provide natural relief for their little ones.

But herbs are not just for treating illnesses – they can also be used to promote better sleep for the whole family. By incorporating calming herbs like chamomile and lavender into your bedtime routine, you can create a peaceful environment that encourages restful nights for everyone.

In addition to promoting better sleep, herbs can also be used for natural skincare and beauty for the family. From soothing sunburns to nourishing dry skin, herbs offer a gentle and effective alternative to harsh chemicals found in many commercial products. By incorporating herbs into your skincare routine, you can promote healthy, glowing skin for the whole family.

If you're interested in incorporating herbs into your daily routine, consider starting an herbal garden at home. Not only is gardening a relaxing and rewarding hobby, but it also allows you to have fresh herbs on hand whenever you need them. By growing your own herbs, you can ensure that your family has access to the highest quality ingredients for better health and wellness.

Overall, embracing a natural lifestyle with herbs can have a positive impact on the mental clarity and focus of the whole family. By incorporating herbs into your daily routine, you can promote better health and wellness for everyone, from the youngest to the oldest family members.

Remember herbs are powerful medications, if you are on any medication by your doctor please see medical assistance before any herbal routine.